HAYFA BERGAOUI
Yessinne Belhaj Taher
IMEN GHADHAB

Teenage pregnancy and childbirth

HAYFA BERGAOUI
Yessinne Belhaj Taher
IMEN GHADHAB

Teenage pregnancy and childbirth

ScienciaScripts

Imprint

Cover image: www.ingimage.com

This book is a translation from the original published under ISBN 978-620-6-71209-1.

Publisher:
Sciencia Scripts
is a trademark of
Dodo Books Indian Ocean Ltd. and OmniScriptum S.R.L publishing group

120 High Road, East Finchley, London, N2 9ED, United Kingdom
Str. Armeneasca 28/1, office 1, Chisinau MD-2012, Republic of Moldova, Europe
Printed at: see last page
ISBN: 978-620-8-26848-0

CONTENTS

INTRODUCTION

For every individual, adolescence and motherhood are periods of transition from the world of childhood to that of adults, from the world of women to that of mothers [1]. The World Health Organisation defines adolescence as the period between the ages of 10 and 19. [2] For psychologists, the definition of adolescence remains imprecise as far as chronological limits are concerned. It is marked by the onset of physical changes (development of secondary sexual characteristics and acquisition of the ability to procreate); there is no coincidence between physical and psychological changes, the latter extending well beyond "physical" puberty [3].Teenage pregnancy raises many questions and remains a public health problem worldwide. In this context, the WHO estimated that in 2012, nearly 16 million girls aged between 15 and 19 gave birth to a child each year, and that these pregnancies are more frequent among adolescents in poor, poorly educated or rural populations [4], and contradictory conclusions have been drawn on the subject [5]. Some studies consider these pregnancies to be at high risk of maternal, obstetric, psychological and neonatal complications, and require effective preventive measures [5-6-7].In fact, these pregnancies appear to be special situations and are a subject of controversy in both industrialised and developing countries. In Tunisia, we are not concerned by this phenomenon, and pregnancies carried to term in adolescents are still a regular occurrence in our maternity units. In an environment dominated by immaturity, irresponsibility, poor socio-economic conditions and sometimes the illegitimacy of pregnancy, the fœto-adolescent prognosis is very poor. maternal life may be clouded [8]. Our work proposes to study this phenomenon in 72 adolescent girls aged under 20 who gave birth at the Monastir maternity and neonatology centre during

2022.The objectives of our study are

1. Study the characteristics socio-economic and cultural of these teenagers
2. Evaluating the quality of prenatal pregnancy monitoring
3. Studying teenage pregnancy and childbirth

To assess the maternal-fetal prognosis and compare our results with those cited in the literature

MATERIALS AND METHODS

This is a retrospective descriptive study based on obstetrical and medical records and operative reports concerning 72 patients aged less than 20 years out of a total of 4487 deliveries carried out in the maternity and neonatology centre of Monastir between 1er January and 31 December 2022. Our choice of the age limit of 19 years was guided by the WHO definition of adolescence. We included all adolescents who gave birth after 22 weeks of amenorrhoea (SA).

I-Sources of information

We searched the birth registers of women under the age of 20 during the study period:

- Maternity ward medical and obstetric records
- Maternity registers
- Surgical reports

II- information sheet

A study form was completed for each parturient and each newborn (**see appendix).**

III-Study statistics

The statistical study and data analysis were processed using SPSS version 13.0.

RESULTS

I-Frequency

During the study period from 1er January to 31 December 2022, we recorded 72 adolescent girls under 20 years of age who gave birth at the Monastir maternity and neonatology centre out of a total of 4487 deliveries, i.e. a frequency of 1.6%.

II- EPIDEMIOLOGICAL CHARACTERISTICS OF ADOLESCENTS

1- Age

We studied the age distribution of adolescent mothers. In our series, the age of the teenage mothers varied between 15 and 19 years, with a majority aged 19 (71.83%), an average age of 18.6

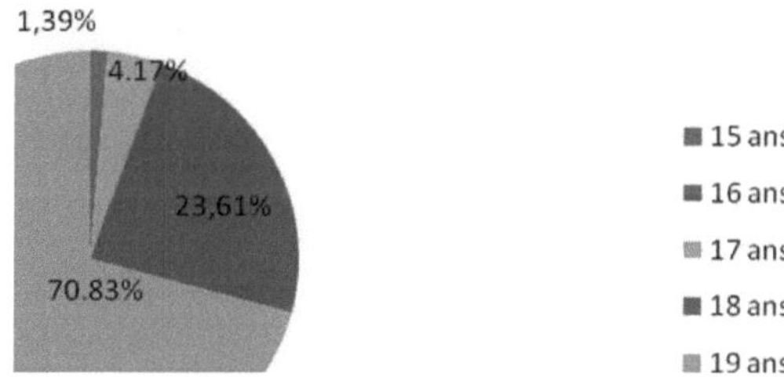

Figure 1: Distribution of teenage girls by age.

2- Origin geographical

Adolescents who have given birth in our maternity unit come mainly from the governorate of Monastir (82%), the majority from the delegation of Moknine (18%) and 18% from other governorates.

Table 1: Breakdown of teenage girls by geographical origin.

Origin	Workforce	percentage
City of Monastir	8	11,11%
Touza	1	1,39%
Ksar hellal	2	2,78%
Moknine	13	18,06%
Teboulba	5	6,94%
Bouhjar	1	1,39%
Khniss	2	2,78%
Werdanine	5	6,94%
Manzel Ennour	8	11,11%
Sidi bannour	1	1,39%
Manzel fares	1	1,39%
Msaken	1	1,39%
Swessi	1	1,39%
Jemmal	5	6,94%
Zeramdine	5	6,94%
Other governorates	13	18,06%
TOTAL	72	100,00%

3- Level education

Adolescents with secondary education accounted for 72.22%, those with primary education for 27.78%. No teenager had completed higher education. There were no cases of illiteracy.

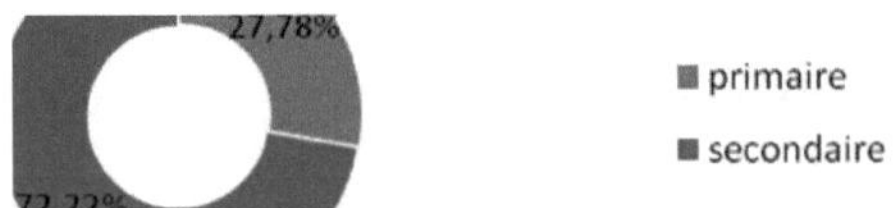

Figure 2: Distribution of adolescent girls by educational level.

4- Marital status

Of the 72 teenage girls, 69 were married, a rate of 95.83%, and 3 were single, representing 4.17% of the total population studied.

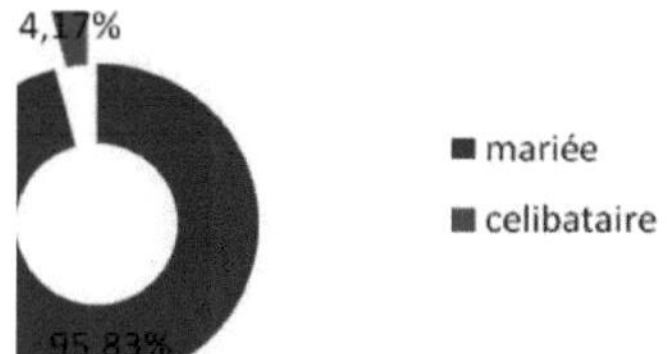

Figure 3: Distribution of teenage girls by marital status.

5- Profession

77.78% of teenage girls have no profession, compared with 20.83% who are blue-collar workers and 1 student (1.39%).

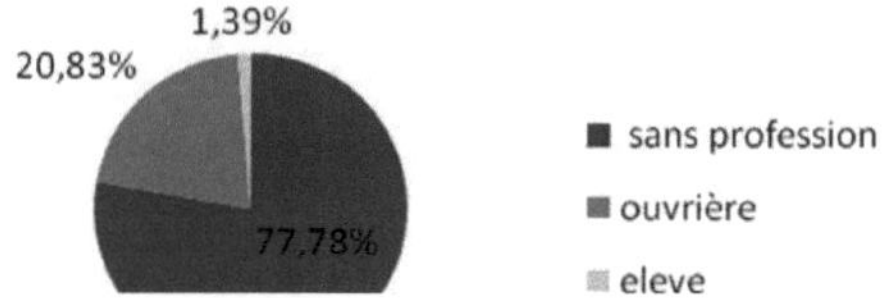

Figure 4: Distribution of teenage girls by profession.

6- Level socio-economic

The majority of teenage girls came from a low socio-economic background, 37.5% from a medium socio-economic background and 5.56% from a high socio-economic background.

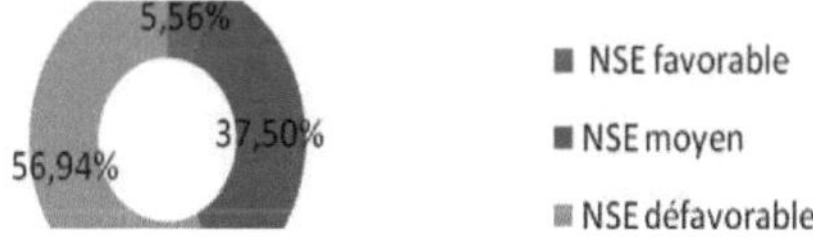

Figure 5: Distribution of teenage girls by socio-economic level.

7- Gestité-parité

Gestité

The average Gestité was 1.24. Adolescent girls included :

Married parturient, aged 19, second gesture, primiparous, undergoing abortion.

An unmarried parturient aged 19, 3rd gesture, primiparous, having undergone 2 abortions.

Married parturient aged 19, 4th procedure, second party having undergone 2 abortions

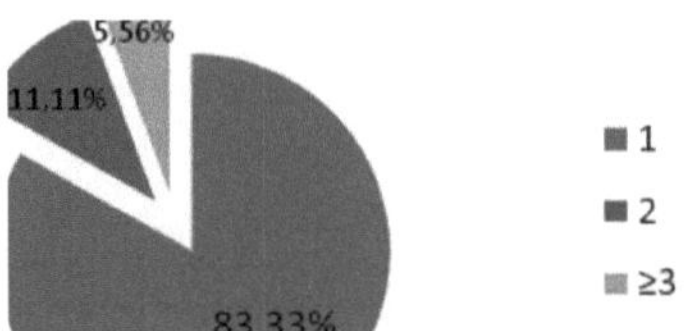

Figure6: Distribution of adolescents by gender.

Parity

The average parity was 1.09; of the 72 deliveries, 65 were primiparous and 7 were second parous.

Figure 7: Distribution of teenage girls by parity.

Multiple pregnancies

In our series there was only one twin pregnancy, which was a mono chorionic bi amniotic pregnancy.

8- History

a. Medical history

In the population studied, some teenage girls had the following medical histories: anaemia, diabetes. Rheumatic fever, heart disease (infundibular IVC, heart failure).

Table 2: Personal medical history of the study population.

		Workforce	Percentage
Pathology	Anemia	2	2.78%
	Infundibular IVC	1	1.39%
	Heart failure	1	1.39%
	RAA	1	1.39%
	Diabetes	1	1.39%
	Hepatic steatosis	1	1,39%
	No pathology	65	90.27%

b. Surgical history

In our sample, there were only 4 appendectomies.

Table 3: Surgical history.

	Workforce	Percentage
Appendectomy	4	5.56%
No intervention	68	94.44%

c. Gynaecological history

Abortion was the most common gynaecological history: 6.94%. 80.56% of adolescents had no notable pathological history.

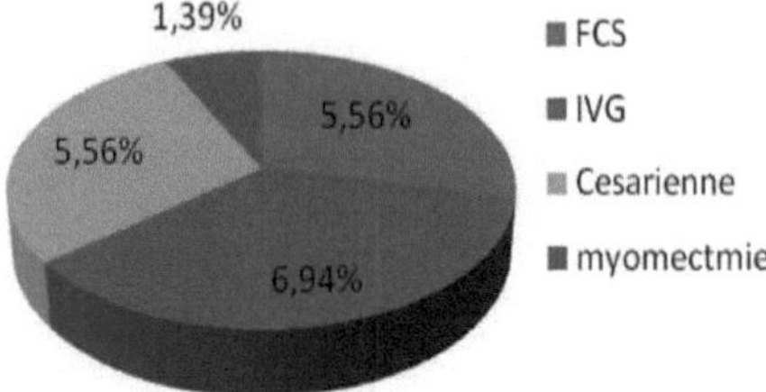

Figure 8: Distribution of adolescents by gynaecological history.

Out of 72 teenagers, only 3 had used a contraceptive method at least once (the pill), compared with 69 who had never tried contraception.

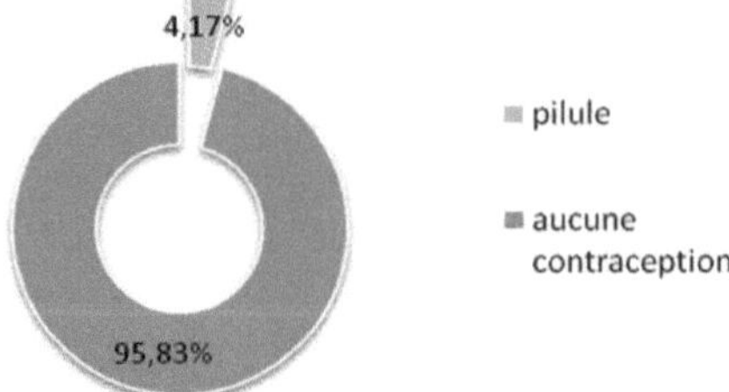

Figure 9: Contraceptive use rates.

10- The spawner

In our series the mean age of the sire was 29.5 years with extremes of 20 to 38 years. The mean age difference between the sire and the mother was 9.7 years, with extremes of 1 to 19 years.

Age of sire

Average age	Age min	Maximum age
29.5 years old	20 years	38 years old

Age difference between sire and dam

Average age difference	Minimum difference	Maximum difference
9.7 years	1	19

III- Pregnancy

1- Prenatal monitoring of pregnancy

19.44% of adolescents did not have the recommended number of ANCs in Tunisia (5 ANC) against 80.56% who had a regularly monitored pregnancy.

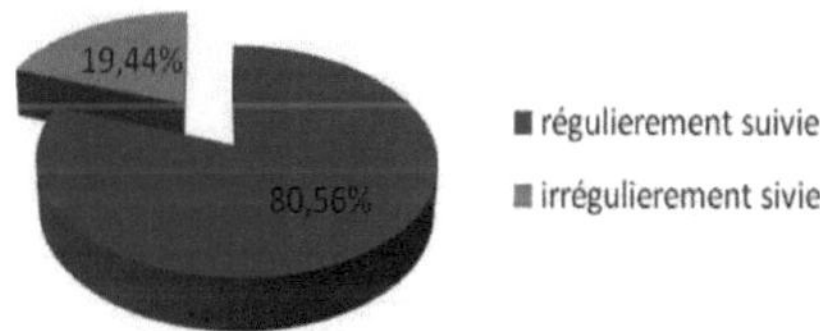

Figure 10: Distribution of teenage girls by prenatal pregnancy follow-up.

2- Term of pregnancy at childbirth

It is difficult to recognise the onset of pregnancy in 3% of married teenagers who do not know the date of their last menstrual period - the approximate ultrasound date was used. The study of the term of pregnancy at delivery revealed :

9 premature deliveries 55 full-term deliveries

7 late-term deliveries 1 overdue delivery

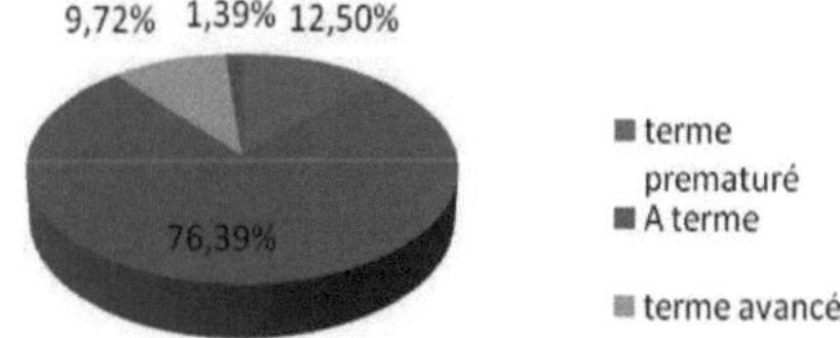

Figure 11: Breakdown of deliveries by term.

3- Possible pathology of pregnancy

Analysis of pregnancy-related pathologies shows that premature rupture of the membranes is the most frequent incident during pregnancy, at a rate of 30.56 %. Anaemia is also frequent at a rate of 26.39% and is generally a pre-existing anaemia that has worsened during pregnancy.

Table 4: Pregnancy-related diseases.

	Workforce	Percentage
Pregnancy-related vomiting	2	2,78%
Anemia	19	26,39%
Thrombocytopenia	2	2,78%
Malformation	1	1,39%
NAP	3	4,17%
Gestational diabetes	7	9,72%
Pregnancy toxaemia	3	4,17%
RPM	22	30,56%
MAP	10	13,89%
Amniotic fluid abnormality	10	13,89%
IUGR	5	6,94%
Macrosomia	4	5,56%
Time limit exceeded	9	12,50%

4- Labour and childbirth

a. Presentations

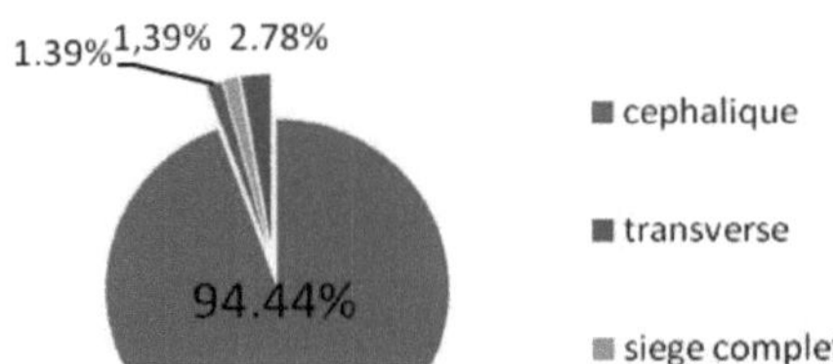

Figure 12: Presentations seen in adolescent girls.

We note that cephalic vertex presentation is the most frequent presentation at a rate of 94.44%, the frequency of breech presentation is

4.17% (1 complete breech + 2 incomplete breech), we also noted a transverse presentation at 1.39%.

b. **Work in progress**

- How to start work

Of a total of 66 parturients for whom the vaginal route was accepted, labour was induced artificially in 11 adolescents.

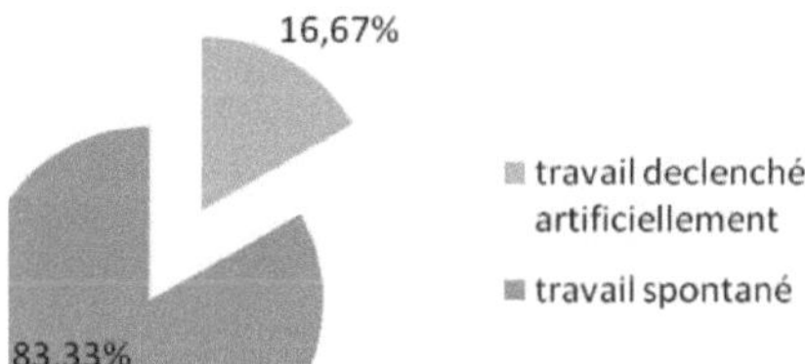

Figure 13: Work entry procedures.

- Indications for labour induction

Labour was induced by an endocervical gel to :

- IUGR: 1 case
- Gestational diabetes: 1 case
- Poorly balanced gravid toxicity: 1 case
- Overrun of term: 1 case
- RPM >12 h: 4 cases

Labour induced by cytotec for RPM with unfavourable bishop: 2 cases

Oxytocin was used in cases of RPM: 4 cases

c. Total working hours

Table 5: Working hours for teenage girls.

	Min	Max	Average
Total working hours	2 hours	20 hours	8.46 hours

The average total working time is 8h.46min, with extremes of 2 hours and 20 hours.

d. Complication of work

- Dynamic and mechanical dystocies

Among the parturients for whom the vaginal route was accepted: 7 adolescents presented with dynamic dystocia
only 1 adolescent presented with mechanical dystocia

- SFA

We observed a rate of 20% of SFA, this anomaly is suspected in the presence of stained amniotic fluid and is objectified by changes in the BDC on the RCF recording.

e. Delivery method

These young mothers include :

56 gave birth by spontaneous vaginal delivery 2 gave birth by instrumental vaginal delivery 6 gave birth by cold Caesarean section 8 by emergency caesarean section

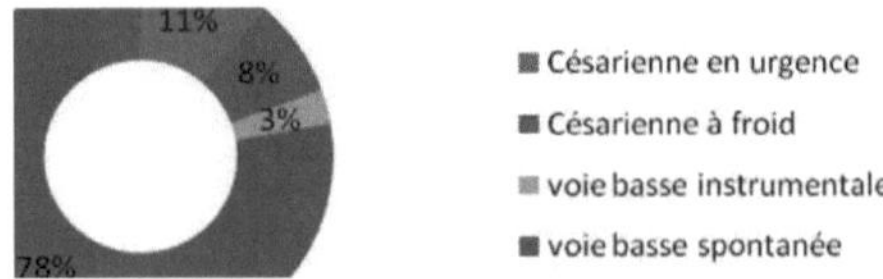

Figure 14: Distribution of adolescents by mode of delivery.

Table 6: Distribution of adolescents according to indication for caesarean section.

Indications for caesarean section		Workforce	%
Prophylactic caesarean section	twin pregnancy+advanced term+unfavourable bishop	1	7,1%
	presentation of seat+primipare	2	14,3%
	frank macrosomia	1	7,1%
	scarred uterus + fresh scar	1	7,1%
	pregnancy toxaemia	1	7,1%
Emergency Caesarean section	Scarred uterus + fresh scar in work	1	7,1%
	heart failure in labour	1	7,1%
	chorioamniotitis	1	7,1%
	RPM+ trip failure	1	7,1%
	RCF pathology	2	14,3%
	procidence of the hand	1	7,1%
	failure of the labour test+RCF pathological	1	7,1%

f. Perineal lesions

• Episiotomy rate

Of the 58 teenagers who gave birth vaginally, 56 had an episiotomy, a rate of almost 97%. Only 2 gave birth without an episiotomy.

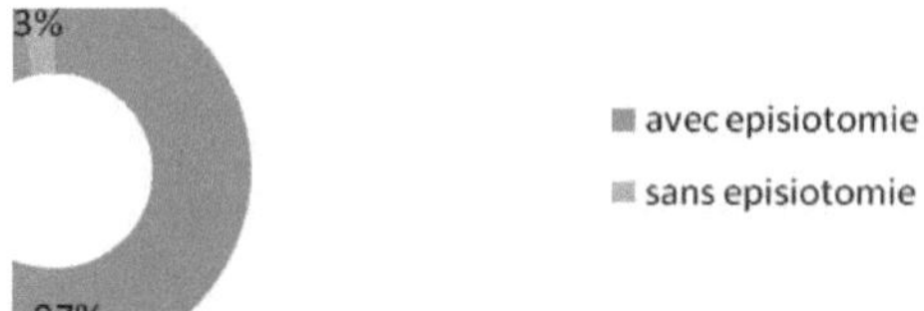

Figure 15: Episiotomy rate.

- Perineal tears

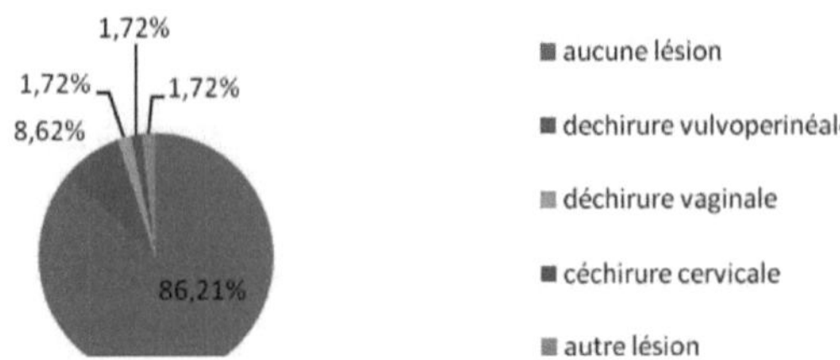

Figure 16: Vulvovaginal and perineal tears during childbirth.

- Episiotomy-tear

3% of teenagers who had an episiotomy suffered a vulvoperineal tear, 3% a vaginal tear, 1% a cervical tear and 1% a ureteral tear. Of the 2 births without episiotomy, one had two tears, one vulvoperineal and one vaginal. This may be closely linked to the lack of preparation for childbirth due to ignorance and a lack of resources for the underprivileged.

5- Delivery

Delivery method

There were two cases of incomplete delivery requiring artificial delivery and uterine revision. Of the 72 cases, 8 cases of haemorrhage in the immediate post-fragment period considered to be of moderate severity, 7 of which were associated with uterine atony and were well controlled by an oxytocin infusion (syntocinon, nalador) and uterine massage, and one haemorrhage due to retained placenta controlled by artificial delivery.

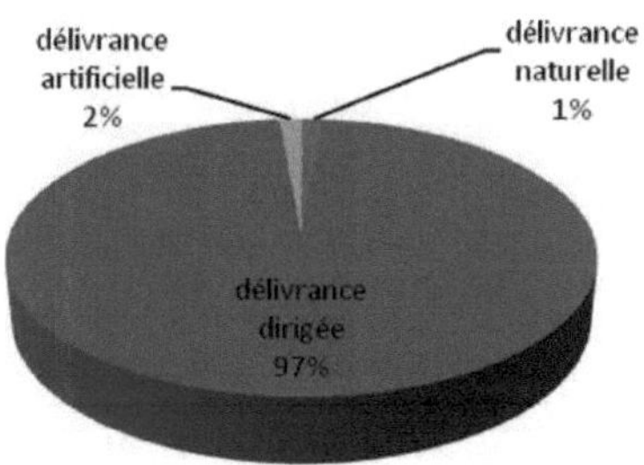

Figure 17: Delivery mode.

6- Aftercare

Length of hospital stay

The average length of hospital stay after vaginal delivery was 2.09 days and 3 days in the case of caesarean section, i.e. an average duration of 2.3 days whatever the method of delivery.

Maternal morbidity

69% of teenagers who gave birth in our department had simple post-natal problems.31% (22) of adolescents experienced post-partum complications.

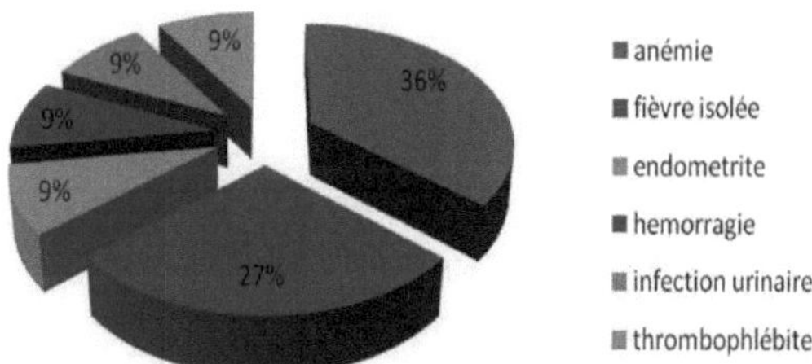

Figure18: Distribution of adolescents according to complications following childbirth.

The most frequent complication was the worsening of anaemia, most often pre-existing during pregnancy. A total of 8 cases of anaemia were noted: 1 case of moderate anaemia, 4 cases of severe anaemia controlled either by venofer treatment or by blood transfusion. The second complication was an isolated fever (6 adolescents) where the patients were put on ATB. There were two cases of post-partum haemorrhage, one of which was recurrent, caused by uterine atony, and the patient was put on nalador with a favourable outcome. In the other case, uterine revision revealed blood clots, so the haemorrhage was controlled by simple revision and uterine massage. Other complications were identified (2 endometritis cases, one of which was haemorrhagic), 2 urinary tract infections, 2 cases of thrombosis of the upper limb where the patients were put on syntron.

IV. Newborn teenager

1. Gender of the child

The predominance of males was 58%.

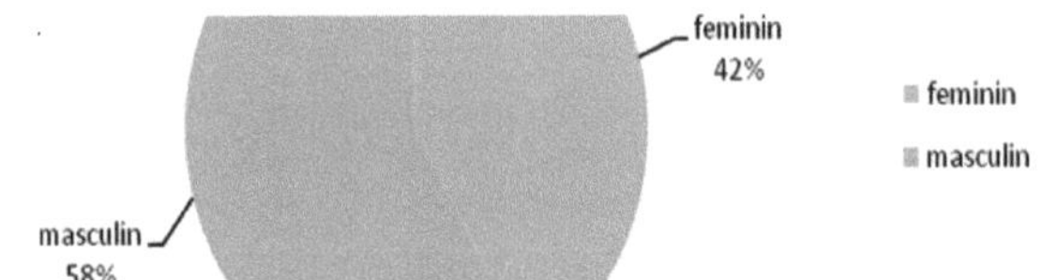

Figure 19: Breakdown of newborn babies by sex.

2. Birth weight

Newborns weighing less than 2,500g are considered low birthweight and those weighing less than 1,500g are considered very low birthweight according to the WHO. The average weight of newborns born to teenage mothers is 3271.53g, with extremes of 720g and 4875g.

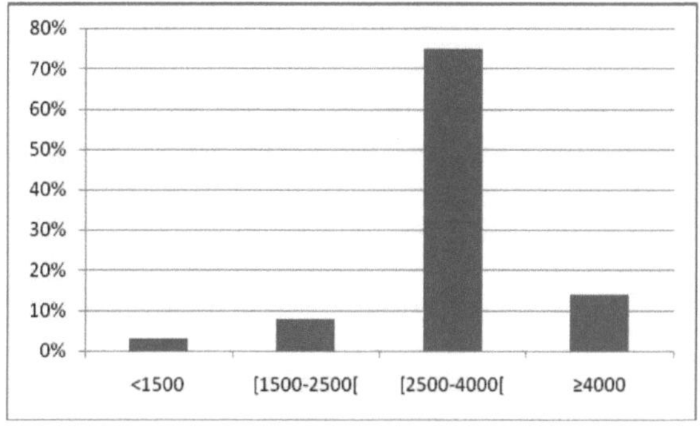

Figure 20: Distribution of newborns according to birth weight.

3. APGAR score

We studied the Apgar score at the first, 5th and tenth minute of life in the newborns of teenage girls

Table 7: Distribution of newborns according to APGAR score.

Apgar score	M1	M5	M10
[0-3]	2	2	2
[4-6]	5	0	0
[7-10]	65	70	70

Neonatal morbidity (APGAR score <7 at M1 of life) is high, and 7 cases were revealed with an Apgar score <7 at the first minute, with one stillborn and one neonate in a state of apparent death.

4. Newborn resuscitation

Light resuscitation was used for 18% of newborns, while heavy resuscitation (ventilation, intubation, transfer to the neonatal intensive care unit) was necessary in 6% of cases.

Resuscitation	Workforce	%
Absent	55	76%
Slight	13	18%
Heavy	4	6%

5. Transfer to neonatology

Out of 73 newborns, 16 were transferred to neonatology after birth.

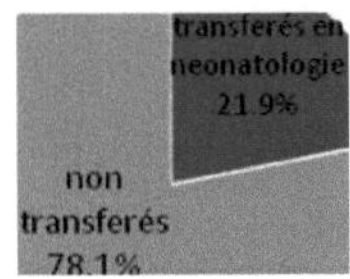

Figure 21: Distribution of newborns by transfer to the neonatology department.

- Indications for transfer to neonatology

Table 8: Indications for transfer to neonatology for newborns born to teenage mothers.

Indication	Workforce	percentage
SFA	4	25,00%
MFI	3	18,75%
DRA	3	18,75%
Prematurity	2	12,50%
Malformation	2	12,50%
DN	1	6,25%
foetal hypertrophy	1	6,25%

6. Fetal anomalies

The following anomalies were found in 3 newborns

- Known cardiac malformation during pregnancy
- Choanes imperméables

- Cryptorchidism

7. Mortality perinatal

In our series we noted 2 cases of perinatal mortality in very premature babies.

V. Breastfeeding

After exclusion of 2 parturients who had their milk supply inhibited by DOSTINEX after the death of their children. 32 mothers practised mixed breastfeeding compared with 30 who preferred exclusive breastfeeding and 8 who chose artificial breastfeeding.

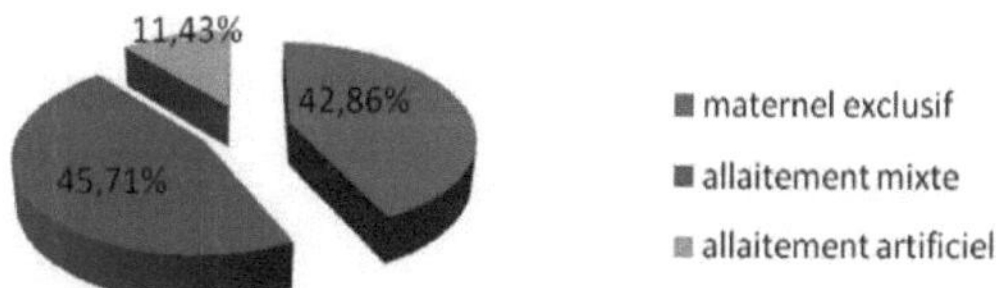

Figure 22: Breastfeeding newborn babies.

DISCUSSION

I. Frequency: incidence

From 1er January to 31 December 2022, we counted 72 teenagers aged between 15 and 19 who gave birth in the gynaecology-obstetrics department of the Monastir maternity and neonatology centre, out of a total of 4,487 deliveries. Among these 72 teenagers, we counted 3 young single mothers, or 4.17% of teenagers. Analysis of the international literature shows variable results depending on the origin and period of the studies, but in all cases the figures are higher than ours.

Table9: Frequency of teenage deliveries in selected foreign series.

authors	Country	study period	age group	TEENAGE BIRTHS (%)
WHO [4]	In the world	2008	15à19	11
Kakudji et al [11]	Lubumbashi (DRC)	2014	<20	2.63
Alouini S et al,[12]	France(Loiret)	2012	10 à19	2.38
L.genest et al [13]	France (Seine saintDenis)	2007 à 2011	12 à 17	1.42
Our series	Tunisia	2022	15 à 19	0,47

II. Characteristics epidemiological

1. Age

The ages of our 72 teenage girls ranged from 15 to 19. The majority were in the 19 age group, with an average age of 18.6.

Table 10: Age of adolescent girls according to Tunisian authors.

Authors	Age groups (years)	Average age (years)
ALA'A SHABANEH [13]	14à19	17,7
EL HAJJ [12]	16à19	17,7
Our series	15à19	18,6

Table 11: Age of adolescent girls according to foreign authors.

Authors	Country	Year	Age range	Average age
GIARDINO [14]	Canada	2008	14à19	17,9
S.alouini et al [12]	France (Loiret department)	2012	10 à 19	16.5
Kakudji luhete et al [11]	Congo(Lubumbashi)	2014	<20	17,6±1.2

2. **Status civil**

The legal age for marriage in Tunisia is 18, according to the Tunisian Marriage Code. personal status [15] In the sample studied, it was found that 69 out of 73 adolescents were married (95.83%) and that the majority had married before the age of 18. Three single mothers (4.17%) were noted, i.e. a rate of 0.47 ‰ in relation to all births. If we compare the rates of unmarried teenage girls in our series and in series from Arab Muslim countries with Western series [11-12-13], we find extremely different rates. This may be explained by the poorly perceived situation of the unmarried pregnant girl due to religious references and the weight of society, which condemn illegitimate relationships.

3. **Socio-economic and cultural profile**

Pregnant teenagers often come from socially, economically or culturally disadvantaged backgrounds.The question arises as to whether early pregnancy is a cultural phenomenon. This observation has been widely taken up by sociologists but also doctors who talk about early marriage and childbearing among young girls as a response to an important cultural dimension. Professor Michel Uzan refers to the concept of "cultural pregnancies", which is very characteristic here: in many African, Eastern European and North African societies, having a child is highly valued. Pregnancy is a rite of passage during which young girls become adult women. Pregnancies are very often planned and expected by a couple or a family [14]. In our series, 72.22% of adolescent girls had dropped out of secondary school, while 27.78% had only attended primary school. The majority belonged to a low socio-economic level (56.94%), compared with 37.50% of medium-level learners and 5.56% from well-off backgrounds. 77.78% of teenage girls have no occupation, compared with 20.83% who are blue-collar workers and 1 student (1.39%).

4. Gynaecological and obstetrical history

The majority of studies show that the rate of primigravida is always dominant [16-14-11-10]. In our series, 83.33% of young mothers were first-time mothers. The average parity was 1.09. The most common gynaecological antecedent was abortion: 6.94%. This may be due to poor contraceptive compliance among adolescents. Among our adolescents, only 3 had used a contraceptive method at least once (the pill), compared with 69 who had never tried contraception.

5. The sire

Fathers are often older than mothers, with an average age of 29.5 years and extremes ranging from 20 to 38 years. The average age difference is 9.7 years. There are few data on the parents of adolescent girls in either the foreign or Tunisian series, perhaps because of the minimal interest shown by the health care team in the spouses of adolescent girls, especially as they are not always present.

III. Pregnancy study

1. Pregnancy follow-up

19.44% of teenage girls did not have the number of ANC recommended in Tunisia (5 ANC) compared with 80.56% who had a regularly monitored pregnancy. In other African countries, it has also been observed that teenage pregnancies are more often poorly monitored than those of adult women [17-18]. This phenomenon is also encountered in developing countries despite the more privileged social context; in 2012 in France, for example, 23.52% had fewer than four prenatal consultations, 41.17% consulted between 4 and 6 times during their pregnancy and 35.29% had more than 7 prenatal consultations [14]. Indeed, the literature tends to show that, overall, pregnancies in minors are less well monitored than adult pregnancies, without any precise distinction being made as to the age of these adolescents[14].

2. Pathologies during pregnancy

According to the WHO, a first pregnancy in a very young girl is risky, and it estimates that while the rate of births to teenagers represents 11% of all births worldwide, it accounts for 23% of the overall burden of morbidity due to pregnancy and childbirth in women of all ages[4]Teenage pregnancy presents increased health risks for the mother, such as anaemia ,hypertension, eclampsia and depressive disorders [19-20], but also for the child's health, including an increased risk of low birth weight, prematurity, depression and, consequently, greater morbidity in childhood[19-21].

RPM

Premature rupture of the membranes before term is the most frequent pathology, complicating approximately 30.56% of pregnancies in our series of adolescents. The frequency of this anomaly can be explained by uterine hypoplasia, the poor prudence of adolescents who are more exposed to trauma, and by the lower infections frequently encountered in this category.

Anemia

In addition to puberty, physical growth and menstrual loss, pregnancy increases iron requirements, which are generally not covered by the diet, and anaemia sets in. In our series, 19 adolescent girls (26.39%) presented with anaemia.

Pregnancy-induced hypertension

Several authors recognise the high frequency of hypertension in very young women and cite biological and endocrine immaturity, primigravida and lack of prenatal monitoring as determining factors in the occurrence of vasculo-renal syndromes. In our series, hypertension was found in only 3 parturients. There were no cases of pre-eclampsia.

Gestational diabetes

In our series we noted 7 cases of GDM, i.e. a rate of 9.72%, with 3 cases of GDM on diet and 4 cases on insulin. Our results contradict those of the literature which state that adolescents are at less risk of developing gestational diabetes because they were more often primiparous and less overweight. Leppalahti et al [21] also found less GDM in adolescents than in adult women, but the differences were not significant.

Prematurity

In our study, 13.89% of pregnancies were complicated by PAD. Other studies have also found a higher rate of prematurity in adolescents [22,23], linked to inadequate perinatal care [24,25] and other associated factors such as smoking, drug addiction and poor socio-economic conditions [13-26]. Scholl et al have shown that becoming pregnant at a young gynaecological age, i.e. starting a pregnancy within two years of menarche, predisposes adolescents to subclinical immaturity of the uterine vasculature, which may be responsible for preterm birth [27].

IV. Labour and delivery

1. Presentations

We note that the cephalic presentation of the vertex is the most frequent 68 at a rate of 94.44%, the frequency of the presentation of the seat is 4.17% (1 complete seat + 2 incomplete seat), we also noted a transverse presentation or 1.39%. Tunisian literature, in line with foreign literature, notes that the young Age has no influence on the type of presentation observed during labour [10].

2. The work

How work starts and how it evolves :

In our series, 83.33% of mothers went into labour spontaneously, compared with 16.76% who went into labour artificially. The most frequent reason for triggering was prolonged RPM with an unfavourable bishop.

- Labour complications

According to Henrion [28] dystocic labour can be explained by :

Uterine hypoplasia can disrupt the progress of labour by causing dynamic dystocia.

*The uterus contracts poorly.

*Dilatation is poor.

Slight pelvic narrowing with fetal-pelvic disproportion can lead to excessive prolongation of labour, which in the absence of intervention can cause fetal distress or death in utero, uterine rupture or vesico-vaginal fistula.

Of the 66 patients for whom the vaginal route was accepted: 7 teenagers had dynamic dystocia

Only 1 adolescent suffered mechanical dystocia. SFA complicated 20% of labours.

3. **Delivery method**

Table 13: Delivery methods according to Tunisian authors.

Authors	Age	Spontaneous V/B	Instrumental extractions	C/S
	(years)	(%)	(%)	(%)
El hajj	<19	76.9%	8.5%	14.6%
Shabeneh	<19	76.3%	8.5%	15.2%
Our series	<20	78%	3%	19%

A higher caesarean section rate was found than in the general population. A study carried out in the DRC between 2013 and 2014 showed that Caesarean sections were significantly more frequent in the under-20s than in the 20-34s [11]. This trend has also been found in other studies [28,29], some of which record a significantly higher rate of caesarean sections in adults, while others find no significant difference.

4. Condition of the perineum

An episiotomy was performed in almost 97% of cases. Only 2 parturients gave birth without an episiotomy. This rate is explained by the absence of perineal preparation for childbirth and therefore the almost systematic practice of episiotomy in primiparous women. The high incidence of tears in teenage girls is explained by the fact that immaturity of the soft tissues with reduced flexibility.

Some publications have found a difference in the rate of intact peins depending on the race of the parturient, the gestational age at the time of delivery and the birth weight of the newborn [30].

V. Post-natal care

In low- and middle-income countries, complications of pregnancy and childbirth are the leading cause of death among women aged 15 to 19 [4].

Complications

The majority (69%) of adolescents delivered in our department had simple post-partum complications. 31% of adolescents experienced post-partum complications. Most authors agree on the benignity and rarity of postpartum complications in adolescents and the absence of significant differences between adolescents and older women [11].

Post-partum hospital stay

The average length of hospital stay after a vaginal delivery is 2.09 days, and 3 days for a caesarean section, i.e. 2.3 days whatever the method of delivery. In France, the average length of hospitalisation after a normal delivery, whatever the age of the adolescent, is 5 days [31] and in

England the length of stay after a normal delivery varies from 6 hours to 2 days [22].

VI. Newborn babies

Studies on teenage pregnancies confirm the competition between the body of the teenage mother and the body of the foetus for nutrients, vitamins and minerals. This explains why teenage girls are twice as likely as adult women to have low-birth-weight babies and more likely to give birth prematurely. [11] In fact, in our series, the average weight of newborn adolescent girls was 3271.53 g. 8 had a birth weight of less than 2500 g, most of whom were premature. The mean weight is in agreement with Tunisian and foreign series [32-33-34-4-5-11-12].

1. Apgar score

We studied the Apgar score at the first, 5th and tenth minute of life in the newborns of adolescent girls. Neonatal morbidity (APGAR score <7 At M1 of life) is severe, we revealed 7 cases with an Apgar score <7 at the first minute with one stillborn and one newborn in a state of apparent death. It should be noted that 44% of premature babies had an APGAR <7 at the first minute of life.

Table 14: Distribution of newborns according to Apgar score in Tunisian series.

Apgar score Authors	<7 in the first minute (%]	<7 at the fifth minute (%)
El hajj	3.7	1.2
Shabeneh	5.1	2.5
Our series	9.7	2.8

Chen [22] found that neonates born to adolescents under the age of 17 had a higher risk of a low Apgar score at 5 minutes. Olausson found that the risk of neonatal and post-neonatal mortality increased steadily with decreasing maternal age [35].

2. Foetal abnormalities

A recent retrospective study carried out in Germany found a higher frequency of chromosomal, cardiac or laproschisis-type malformations in the adolescent population [36].

The following anomalies were found in newborns

- Known heart defects during pregnancy
- Waterproof shawls
- Cryptorchidism

3. Transfer to neonatology

In our series, the rate of transfer to neonatology was 21.9%. The main reason for transfer was SFA (25%), followed by suspected IMF and ARD (18.75%), and finally prematurity and malformations (12.5%). Most authors [37-38- 7- 39] have found that the rate of transfer to neonatology is significantly higher in adolescents than in control groups. This may be explained by the high incidence of RPM, which most often leads to premature delivery, and by MFI, which is also favoured by RPM.

4. Perinatal mortality

A study carried out by Foueliack in Cameroon found a risk of perinatal mortality twice as high in adolescents as in the adult population. These results are consistent with numerous studies [40].
In our series we noted 2 cases of neonatal death.

VII. Breastfeeding

From a biological point of view, lactation is perfectly possible in teenage girls. After exclusion of 2 parturients whose milk supply was inhibited by DOSTINEX after the death of their children. 32 mothers practised mixed breastfeeding compared with 30 who preferred exclusive breastfeeding and 8 who chose artificial breastfeeding. According to the CPNP report, teenage girls, single mothers and women with less education or low incomes appear to be more likely to breastfeed their babies than women in similar situations in the general population [41].

RECOMMENDATIONS

When it comes to teenage pregnancy, many current and scholarly publications list the difficulties faced by a young mother and her child. To prevent these pregnancies, the who [4] has issued a number of recommendations on actions to be taken and research to be undertaken to prevent early pregnancies and their negative repercussions on reproductive health.

i. REDUCE THE NUMBER OF MARRIAGES BEFORE THE AGE OF 18 :

-Political leaders must adopt and implement laws that

prohibit marriage before the age of 18

-Individuals, families and communities must :

- Keeping girls in school: girls who attend school are less likely to be

to be married are too young. Getting girls into school has a positive impact on their health and that of their children.

- influence the social norms that support early marriage

ii. EDUCATING TEENAGERS ABOUT THEIR SEXUALITY

It is therefore recommended to carry out :

i. Prevention programmes based on educational activities in the form of role-playing, video screenings and discussion groups addressing these themes should be developed in schools, particularly those with more vulnerable populations. They would also help to strengthen links between peers and provide social and emotional support. The WHO affirms that these programmes must be linked to contraceptive advice and dispensing structures, given that young girls who have experienced pregnancy have a false knowledge of contraception and misuse it:

iii. Enable teenagers to access contraceptive services; Teenagers often do not seek contraceptive services because they are afraid of social stigmatisation or being judged by medical staff. Health systems must be able to respond better to the needs of adolescents and be more welcoming.

iv. INCREASE THE USE OF SKILLED CARE DURING PREGNANCY, CHILDBIRTH AND THE POSTNATAL PERIOD:

- Inform teenage girls and members of their

communities on the importance of qualified care during pregnancy, childbirth and the postnatal period: (It is important to disseminate accurate information on the risks associated with a lack of access to qualified care, both for the mother and the baby, and to indicate where such care can be obtained)

- An ultrasound scan during the first trimester is recommended.

recommended not only for adequate dating of pregnancy and assessment of increased risk of preterm delivery

Prepare the young mother-to-be and her partner and parents for birth and obstetric emergencies: Pregnant teenagers must receive the support they need to be well prepared for birth and obstetric emergencies, in particular by having a birth plan. Preparation for birth and the risks of obstetric emergencies should be an integral part of antenatal care: Fathers and partners should be involved in antenatal classes.

CONCLUSION

Adolescence refers to a period of growth necessary to achieve adult status. It is a long process, the beginning of which is marked by puberty. It is not only characterised by the typical physical changes; it is a time of life full of emotional and psychological transformations that are just as important as those of a physical nature. Adolescents are questioning their identity and feel a growing need for independence, which they find in pregnancy. There is a certain value placed on motherhood, with motherhood representing the transition to the social status of woman, and pregnancy being the path that leads to femininity, the adolescent-mother-woman trinity. As a result, the phenomenon of teenage pregnancy has been the subject of numerous studies and contradictory conclusions have been drawn; some studies consider teenage pregnancies to be high-risk pregnancies with maternal, obstetric, psychological and neonatal complications, requiring effective and widespread preventive measures. Others are much less alarmist.The aims of our retrospective study were to: Study the socio-economic and cultural characteristics of these teenagers Assess the quality of prenatal pregnancy monitoring Studying teenage pregnancy and childbirth To evaluate the maternal-fetal prognosis and compare our results with those cited in the literatureWe recorded 72 patients aged under 20 years out of a total of 4,487 deliveries at the Monastir maternity and neonatology centre over the period 1er January to 31 December 2022, **i.e. a frequency of 1.6%.** In our series, the age of the teenage mothers varied between 15 and 19 years, with an average age of 18.6 years. Most of the young mothers had no occupation. The average age of the sire was 29.5 years, with extremes of 20 and 38 years.The average age difference between sire and dam was 9.7 years. The majority of the mothers were primigravida. The mean Gestité was 1.24 and the mean parity 1.09. 6.94% had a history of abortion and 5.56% had had a miscarriage. Of the 72 adolescents, only 3 had been put on contraception (pill) at least once (4.17%). 19.44% of teenagers were not properly monitored during pregnancy Analysis of pregnancy-related pathologies shows that premature rupture of the membranes is the most frequent incident during pregnancy. Anaemia is also frequent, and is generally a pre-existing anaemia that has been aggravated by pregnancy. Labour in adolescents appears to be rather physiological, with most of them going into labour spontaneously. 55 mothers gave birth at full term, compared with 9 who gave birth at premature term and 8 at prolonged term. 81% of patients gave birth by natural route and 19% by caesarean section. In the case of vaginal delivery, the episiotomy rate was 97%. Out of 72 cases, there were 8 cases of immediate post-partum haemorrhage of moderate severity with a favourable outcome. The average length of hospital stay is 2.3 days, irrespective of the route of treatment. Delivery The post-partum period was uncomplicated for 69% of women. 31% experienced post-partum complications, mainly anaemia, which was already present and was exacerbated by the birth losses. The average weight of newborn teenage mothers is 3271.53 g. In studying the Apgar score, we noted 7 cases with a score of less than 7 at the first minute. Out of 73 newborns, 16 were transferred to neonatology after birth. There were 2 cases of perinatal mortality in very premature babies. In total, our population does not appear to be at high risk, as mentioned in certain studies, but it is imperative to improve the quality of prenatal care in terms of reinforcing pregnancy monitoring in order to identify high-risk situations at an early stage so that they can benefit from optimal care and give birth under optimal conditions.

BIBLIOGRAPHY

Sylvain bisleau. quand la maternite rencontre l'adolescence :des enjeux psychiques aux enjeux du soin. thesis de medecine.Nante 2012N°119.

Adolescent Health Committee (Canadian Paediatric Society - CPS), The age limit between adolescence and adulthood. Pediatrics&Child health 2003 ;8(9) :578].

Rotten D., GEMIGON O. contraception et sexualite:particularite liees a l'adolescence.Rev.Prat.(paris),1989;39:4

World Health Organization. Early marriage, teenage pregnancy and young women. Sixty-fifth World Health Assembly. Item 13.4 of the provisional agenda; 2012

Soula O., CARIES G., Largeaud M., El Guindi W., Montoya Y. Pregnancy and childbirth in adolescents under 15 J Gyriecol Obstet Biol Reprod 2006; 35 :53-61

Dedecker F, De Bailliencourt T, Barau G et al. Etude des facteurs de risques obstetricaux dans le suivi de 365 grossesses primipares adolescentes l'ile de la Reunion. J Gynecol. Obstet. Biol.de la Reproduction Volume 34, ISSUE7, PART 1,November 2005,649-701

Lloki H., KOUBAKA R., ITOUA c., MBEMBA Moutounou G., M. adolescent pregnancy and childbirth in the Congo Gynecol Obstet Biol Reprod 2004 ; 33,1 :37-42

M.BELKHERI, S.NADOU, D.ZIAN, A.LAKHDAR, A.CHAOUI. TEENAGE PREGNANCY AND CHILDBIRTH. LES CAHIERS DU MEDECIN. TOME VII, N°77. NOVEMBER 2004

EL HAJJ M. PREGNANCY AND CHILDBIRTH IN ADOLESCENTS UNDER 19 YEARS OF AGE, 82 CASES. THESIS DE MEDECINE.SFAX2007

Shabaneh a. Pregnancy and childbirth in adolescents under 19 years of age ANS, A PROPOS DE 118 CAS. THESIS DE

MEDECINE.MONASTIR 2010 N°.
Kakudji I , oivier m, albert m , etude de pronostic maternet au cours de l'accouchement chez l'adolescente a lubumashi ,republique democratique du congo,vol9,2017,3 ;4
Alouini S, et alRisk factors in adolescent pregnancy, childbirth and postpartum in the Loiret department. J Gynecol Obstet Biol Reprod2014;8
Genest L, Decroix H, Rotten D, Simmat-Durand L. Earlymotherhood: sociodemographic profiles of 220 teenage mothers in Seine-Saint-Denis. J Gynecol Obstet Biol Reprod2014;43:351-60.
GIARDINO J,GONZALEZ A,STEINER M,ET AL.EFFECTS OF MOTHERHOOD ON PHYSIOLOGICAL AND SUBJECTIVE RESPONSES TO INFANT CRIES IN TEENAGE MOTHERS: A COMPARISON WITH NON-MOTHERS AND ADULT MOTHERS.HORM BEHAV.2008 JAN;53(1):149-58
PERSONAL STATUS CODE
MESBAHI, PR.A.CHAOUI, PR.FARHATI Teenage pregnancy and childbirth: characteristics and profile (about 122 cases).
Tandu-Umba NF, Yanga K, Mputu L. Profil obstetrical de la maternite precoce a Kinshasa (Zaïre). J Gyn Obstet BiolReprod1983; 12: 873-7
Ba MG, Moreau JC, Cisse ML, Dotou C, Bah MD, Diadhiou F.Les particularites obstetricales de la maternite precoce auCHU de Dakar (À propos de 1 360 cas). Burkina Medical1998; 2: 5-8.9. Djanhan Y, Kodjo R, Gondo D, Abauleth YR, Bohoussou K
Tandu-Umba NF, Yanga K, Mputu L. Profil obstetrical de la maternite precoce a Kinshasa (Zaïre). J Gyn Obstet BiolReprod1983; 12: 873-7
Ba MG, Moreau JC, Cisse ML, Dotou C, Bah MD, Diadhiou F.Les particularites obstetricales de la maternite precoce auCHU de Dakar (À propos de 1 360 cas). Burkina Medical1998; 2: 5-8.9. Djanhan Y, Kodjo R, Gondo D, Abauleth YR, Bohoussou K

Leppälahti S, Gissler M, Mentula M, Heikinheimo O. Is tee-nage pregnancy an obstetric risk in a welfare society? Apopulation-based study in Finland, from 2006 to 2011. BMJ Open 2013;3:e003225

CHEN XK, Wen SW, Fleming N, et al. Teenage pregnancy andadverse birth outcomes: a large population based retrospectivecohort study. Int J Epidemiol 2007;36:368-73.

Malabarey OT, Balayla J, Klam SL, et al. Pregnancies in young adolescent mothers: a population-based study on 37 million births. J Pediatr Adolesc Gynecol 2012;25:98-102.

Karabulut A, Ozkan S, Bozkurt AI, Karahan T, Kayan S. Perinataloutcomes and risk factors in adolescent and advanced age pregnancies: comparison with normal reproductive age women. JObstet Gynaecol 2013;33:346-50.

Guiot O, Foucan T, Janky E, Kadhel P. Pregnancies among underage girls in Guadeloupe: a new inventory. J Gynecol Obstet BiolReprod 2013;42:372-82

Ekwoo EE, Moawad A. Maternal age and preterm birth in a black population. Paediatr Perinat Epidemiol 2000;14:145-51.

Scholl TO, Hediger ML, Salmon RW, Belsky DH, Ances IG. Association between low gynaecological age and preterm birth. Paediatr Perinat Epidemiol 1989;3:357-66.

Henrion r . mutilations genitales feminines, mariages forces et grossesse precoces.bull.acad.natle med,2003,187n°6.

Ayuba II, Gani O. Outcome of teenage pregnancy in the Niger delta of NIGERIA. ETHIOP J HEALTH SCI. 2012; 22(1): 45-50.

VENDITELLI F.,GALLOT D. WHAT ARE THE EPIDEMIOLOGICAL DATA CONCERNING EPISIOTOMY.J.GNECOL.OBSTET.BIOL.REPROD 2006:35(SUPPL.AN01):1S12-1S23.

VATRIN E.,FONTAINE A.,LAMBA P.,ENGELMANN P.DUREE DU

SEJOUR EN MATERNITE APRES UN ACCOUCHEMENT NORMAL.J.GYNECOL.OBSTET.BIOL.REPROD 2000 ;29 :94-101Bouajilla M. la grossesse chez l'adolescente.thesis de medecine.tunis1987N°195

mhenni h. grossesse et accouchement chez l'adolescente. thesis de medecine. Monastir 1995.n°260

FELLAH M. PREGNANCY AND CHILDBIRTH IN ADOLESCENT GIRLS UNDER 20 ANS. THÈSE DE MEDECINE.TUNIS 1999.N°86

Olausson PO, Cnattingius S, Haglund B. Teenage pregnancies and risk of late fetal death and infant mortality. British Journal of Obstetrics and Gynaecology. 1999; 106: 116-121. Google Scholar

Eckmann-Scholz C, von Kaisenberg CS, Alkatout I, Jonat W, Rajabi-Wieckhorst A. Pathologic ultrasound findings and risk for congenital anomalies in teenage pregnancies. J Matern Fetal Neonatal Med 2012;25:1950-2

CARLES G.,JACQUELIN X.,RAYNAL P.,BETSCH M.,ZOCCARATO A.-M PREGNANCY AND CHILDBIRTH IN TEENAGE GIRLS UNDER 16 ANS.J.GYNECOL.OBSTET.BIOL REPROD.1998 ;27 :508-513

COLLIN O. GROSSESSE ET ACCOUCHEMENT CHEZ L'ADOLESCENTE DE MOINS DE 16 ANS EN GUYANE.THESE DE MEDECINE.NANCY 2000 N°65

MAYANDA H.F.,MALONGA H., DJOUOB S., NZINGOULA S. NOUVEAU-NES DE MERES ADOLESCENTES AU CONGO.REV.DE PED.,T.XXVI, NOVEMBER 1999, P.307-314

Fouelifack FY, Tameh TY, Mbong EN, Nana PN, Fouedjio JH, Fouogue JT, Mbu RE. Outcome of deliveries among adolescent GIRLS AT the Yaoundé central hospital. BMC Pregnancy Childbirth. 2014 Mar 17; 14: 102.HEALTH CANADA.CANADIAN PRENATAL NUTRITION PROGRAM.1998 QIC REPORT.

APPENDIX

Study sheet

I. Identification

II. Origin

1. City of Monastir
2. Monastir Delegation
3. Other governorates

III. Age

IV. Age of spouse

V. **Civil status**

1. Married
2. Single
3. Other

VI. Level of education

1. Primary
2. Secondary
3. Superior
4. Illiterate

VII. Profession

VIII. Socio-economic level

1. Low
2. Medium
3. Easy

IX. Antecedents

1. Medical
2. Surgical
3. Gynaecological

- DPR

- Gestité
- Parity
- Abortion
- ABORTION
- Other...

X. Contraception

1. No
2. Yes

- Pill
- IUD
- Other

XI. Current pregnancy

1. DDR
2. Type of pregnancy
3. Number of NPCs
4. Preparing for childbirth

- Yes
- No

5. Pregnancy-related pathology

- No pathology
- Urinary tract infection
- Anemia
- Pregnancy-induced hypertension/pre-eclampsia
- Gestational diabetes
- RPM
- MAP
- IUGR
- Amniotic fluid abnormality
- Term advanced/exceeded
- Other

XII. Labour and delivery

1. Work

a. How to start work

- Spontaneous
- Prostaglandins
- Oxytocin

b. Total working hours

c. Labour complications

- Dynamic dystocia
- Mechanical dystocia
- SFA

d. Presentation during work

- Cephalic
- Seat
- Transverse

2. Birth

a. Mode

- Spontaneous vaginal delivery
- Instrumental bass voice
- Scheduled caesarean section

➔Indication(s)

- Emergency Caesarean section

➔Indication(s)

b. Term of pregnancy to delivery

- Eventually
- Premature term
- Past due date

c. Episiotomy

- Yes

- No

d. Perineal lesions

- No
- Vagina
- Rectum
- Collar
- Other...

3. Delivery

a. Mode

- Spontaneous
- Directed
- Artificial

b. Placenta

- Full
- Incomplete

c. Immediate post-partum haemorrhage

- No
- Yes

Control and development

XIII. Post-natal care

1. Simple suites
2. Complicated sequels

- Isolated fever
- Infections
- Endometritis
- Anemia
- Thrombophlebitis
- Other

3. Length of hospital stay

XIV. Newborn

1. Gender
2. Weight
3. Apgar

- M1
- M5
- M10

4. Resuscitation

- Absent
- Slight
- Heavy

5. Transfer to neonatology

a. Yes

- Indication(s)

b. No

6. Perinatal mortality Breastfeeding

1. Exclusive maternal
2. Mixed
3. Artificial

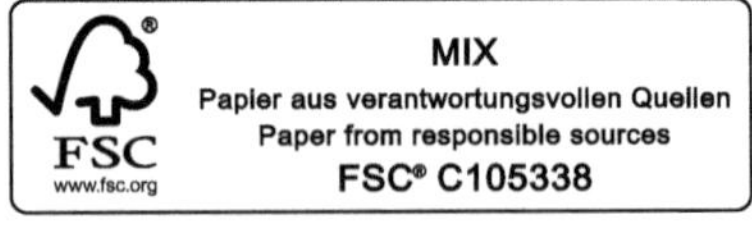

Printed by Books on Demand GmbH, Norderstedt / Germany